MEDITERRANEAN DIET FOR TYPE 2 DIABETICS

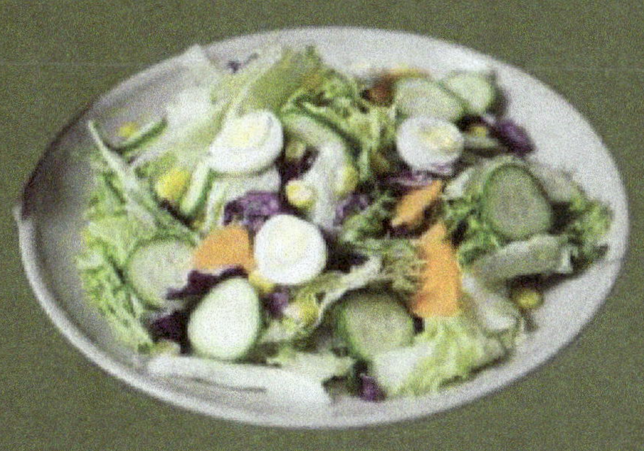

AASHVI DHINGRA

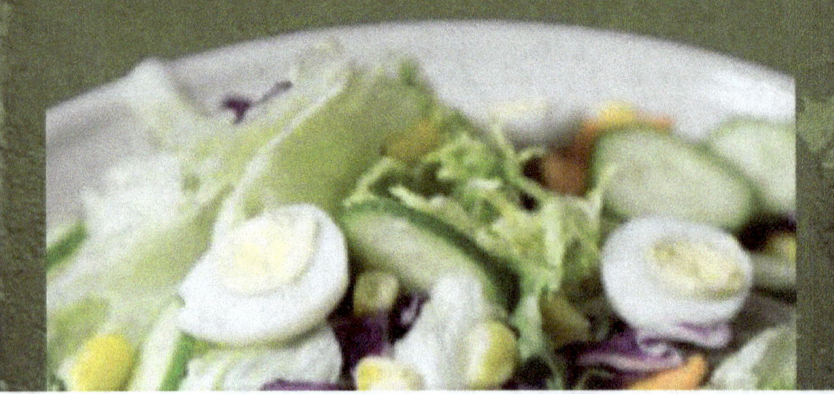

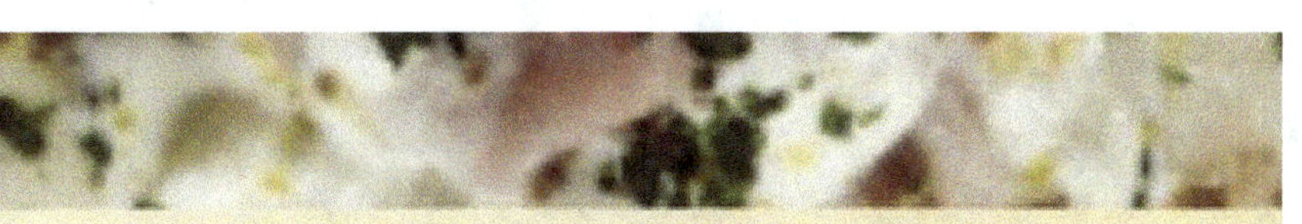

Type 2 diabetes, a chronic metabolic disorder characterized by elevated blood glucose levels, affects millions of people worldwide. The prevalence of this condition has been on the rise, largely attributed to modern lifestyles, sedentary habits, and poor dietary choices. However, there is growing evidence that adopting a Mediterranean diet, rich in diverse and flavorful foods inspired by various cultures, can play a crucial role in managing, preventing, and even reversing type 2 diabetes.

The Mediterranean diet, renowned for its association with lower rates of cardiovascular disease, obesity, and diabetes, is not a modern-day fad. It has its roots in the traditional dietary patterns of countries bordering the Mediterranean Sea, such as Greece, Italy, Spain, and other North African and Middle Eastern regions. Research has consistently shown that adherence to this diet is linked to a reduced risk of type 2 diabetes, as well as improved glycemic control for those already diagnosed with the condition.

A MULTICULTURAL RECIPES FOR REVERSING AND PREVENTING TYPE 2 DIABETES

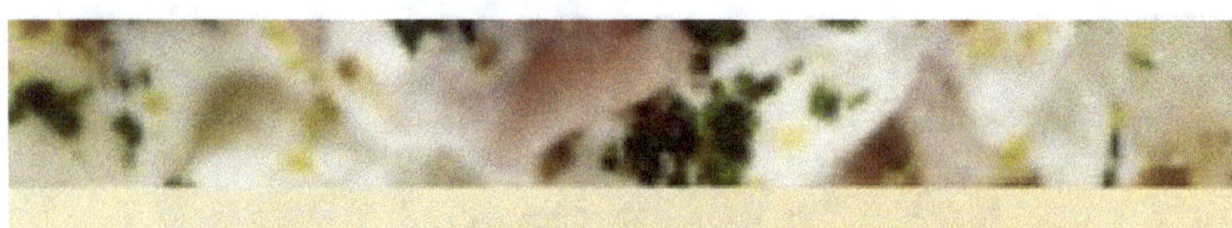

So, what makes the Mediterranean diet so uniquely beneficial for individuals living with type 2 diabetes? The answer lies in its holistic and balanced approach to nutrition, incorporating an abundance of nutrient-dense, whole foods while minimizing processed and sugary options. The diet emphasizes fresh fruits and vegetables, whole grains, legumes, nuts, seeds, and heart-healthy fats, primarily from olive oil. Meanwhile, it discourages the excessive consumption of red meat, refined sugars, and processed foods, which are known to exacerbate diabetes symptoms and complications.

Moreover, one of the key strengths of the Mediterranean diet is its versatility and adaptability to a multitude of cultural cuisines. Emphasizing the inclusion of various regional flavors, herbs, and spices, the Mediterranean diet can be effortlessly tailored to suit the palates and dietary preferences of people from diverse backgrounds. By integrating multicultural recipes into the Mediterranean diet framework, individuals with type 2 diabetes can enjoy a wide array of delicious dishes that cater to their unique cultural tastes.

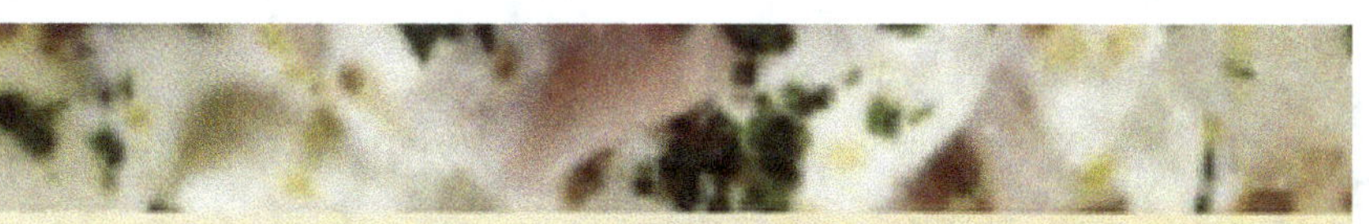

This book, "Mediterranean Diet for Type 2 Diabetics: A Multicultural Collection of Recipes for Reversing and Preventing Type 2 Diabetes," aims to serve as a comprehensive guide, empowering readers to take charge of their health through the adoption of a healthful and enjoyable dietary regimen. By delving into the scientific evidence supporting the efficacy of the Mediterranean diet for diabetes management, we seek to provide a solid foundation for understanding the rationale behind this lifestyle choice.

The chapters in this book will walk you through the fundamental principles of the Mediterranean diet, breaking down the key components of this heart-healthy way of eating. You will discover the nutritional benefits of incorporating fresh, seasonal produce, lean proteins, and beneficial fats, all of which contribute to improved blood sugar control and overall well-being.

A MULTICULTURAL RECIPES FOR REVERSING AND PREVENTING TYPE 2 DIABETES

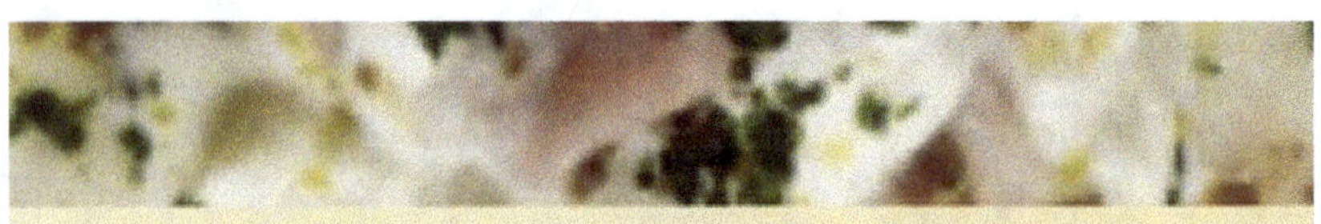

Additionally, this book celebrates the rich culinary diversity of the Mediterranean region and beyond. By exploring traditional recipes from various cultures, we hope to inspire you to explore new flavors and embrace multicultural cuisine, all while ensuring these recipes are tailored to meet the dietary needs of individuals living with type 2 diabetes.

Each chapter contains carefully curated recipes, meticulously designed to be diabetes-friendly, easy to prepare, and, above all, delicious. From breakfast delights to nourishing dinners, sides and snacks to delectable desserts, we have compiled a diverse assortment of dishes that you can enjoy without compromising on taste or nutrition.

Kindly leave a review on Amazon. It will help us improve on future publications. Thanks

A MULTICULTURAL RECIPES FOR REVERSING AND PREVENTING TYPE 2 DIABETES

ACKNOWLEDGEMENT

Writing this book on "Diabetic Diet: Delicious and Mediterranean Recipes from Around the World" has been a rewarding journey, and I am deeply grateful to all those who supported and contributed to its creation. The realization of this project would not have been possible without the collective effort and expertise of several individuals whom I would like to express my heartfelt gratitude to:

Special recognition goes to the individuals who generously shared their cultural recipes and culinary knowledge, making this book a truly diverse and enriching collection of Mediterranean and Diabetic friendly dishes from various parts of the world. Their willingness to contribute and collaborate made this book unique and vibrant.

INTRODUCTION

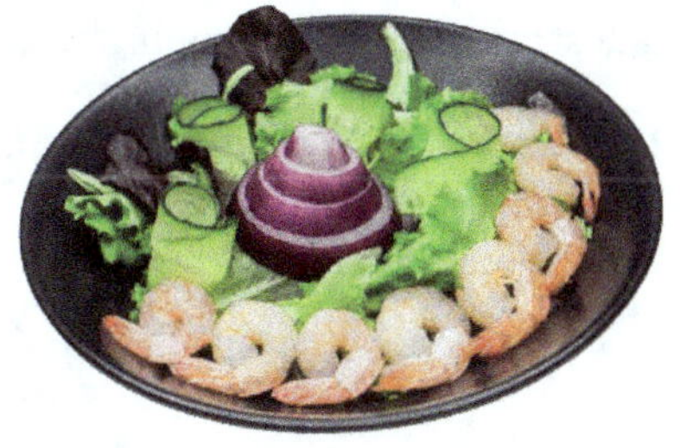

1.1 Understanding Type 2 Diabetes

Type 2 diabetes is a chronic metabolic disorder characterized by high levels of blood sugar (glucose) resulting from the body's inability to properly utilize insulin or produce enough of it. Insulin is a hormone that regulates blood sugar levels by facilitating the absorption of glucose into cells for energy production. When the body becomes resistant to insulin or fails to produce sufficient amounts of it, glucose accumulates in the bloodstream, leading to hyperglycemia.

Several factors contribute to the development of type 2 diabetes, including genetics, sedentary lifestyle, obesity, and poor dietary habits. Unlike type 1 diabetes, which is an autoimmune condition where the body's immune system attacks and destroys insulin-producing cells in the pancreas, type 2 diabetes is often preventable and manageable through lifestyle changes, especially diet and exercise.

1.2 The Mediterranean Diet Approach

The Mediterranean diet is a traditional eating pattern inspired by the dietary habits of people living in countries bordering the Mediterranean Sea, such as Greece, Italy, Spain, and Southern France. It has gained immense popularity worldwide due to its numerous health benefits and its potential to combat chronic diseases like type 2 diabetes.

The main components of the Mediterranean diet include:

1. Abundant Plant-Based Foods: This diet emphasizes a high consumption of fruits, vegetables, whole grains, legumes, nuts, and seeds. These foods are rich in fiber, vitamins, minerals, and antioxidants, which can help reduce inflammation and improve insulin sensitivity.

2. Healthy Fats: The Mediterranean diet is not a low-fat diet; rather, it promotes the consumption of healthy fats primarily from sources like olive oil, nuts, and fatty fish. These fats are high in monounsaturated and omega-3 fatty acids, which have been shown to support heart health and improve insulin function.

3. Moderate Protein: The diet includes moderate amounts of protein from sources like fish, poultry, dairy, and legumes. Adequate protein

intake is essential for maintaining muscle mass and promoting satiety.

4. Reducing Red Meat and Sweets: Red meat and sweets are limited in the Mediterranean diet. This reduction in red meat consumption may be particularly beneficial for individuals with type 2 diabetes, as it can help control blood sugar levels and reduce the risk of cardiovascular complications.

5. Red Wine (in moderation): Some versions of the Mediterranean diet include moderate consumption of red wine with meals. The antioxidants found in red wine, such as resveratrol, have been associated with potential health benefits, but excessive alcohol consumption should be avoided.

1.3 Benefits of the Mediterranean Diet for Type 2 Diabetics

The Mediterranean diet has garnered attention from researchers and healthcare professionals due to its positive impact on type 2 diabetes management. Some of the notable benefits include:

- Improved Blood Sugar Control: The Mediterranean diet's emphasis on whole grains, fruits, vegetables, and healthy fats can help stabilize blood sugar levels and reduce insulin resistance. By promoting better glucose regulation, it aids in managing diabetes and reducing the risk of complications.

- Enhanced Heart Health: Individuals with type 2 diabetes are at a higher risk of developing cardiovascular issues. The Mediterranean diet's focus on heart-healthy fats, such as those found in olive oil and fatty fish, can help lower bad cholesterol levels (LDL) and reduce the risk of heart disease.

- Weight Management: Obesity is a significant risk factor for type 2 diabetes. The Mediterranean diet's nutrient-dense, high-fiber foods can help individuals achieve and maintain a healthy weight, which is essential for diabetes management.

- Reduced Inflammation: Chronic inflammation plays a role in the development and progression of type 2 diabetes. The Mediterranean diet's abundance of antioxidants from fruits, vegetables, and olive oil can help combat inflammation, thus potentially reducing the severity of diabetes and its complications.

- Lower Risk of Diabetes Complications: Type 2 diabetes can lead to various complications, such as nerve damage, kidney disease, and eye problems. The Mediterranean diet's nutrient-rich foods provide essential vitamins and minerals that support overall health and can reduce the risk of these complications.

- Satiety and Sustainable Eating: The Mediterranean diet is not a restrictive or fad diet but rather promotes a balanced and sustainable approach to eating. Its inclusion of healthy fats, protein, and fiber-rich foods can help individuals feel fuller for longer, reducing the urge to overeat or indulge in unhealthy snacks, which is crucial for individuals with diabetes managing their blood sugar levels.

- Better Blood Pressure Management: High blood pressure often accompanies type 2 diabetes, increasing the risk of cardiovascular events. The Mediterranean diet's emphasis on foods that support heart health, such as leafy greens, nuts, and fish, can help manage blood pressure levels effectively.

- Positive Effect on Insulin Resistance: Insulin resistance is a hallmark of type 2 diabetes. The Mediterranean diet has been shown to improve insulin sensitivity, making it easier for the body to use insulin effectively and regulate blood sugar levels more efficiently.

- Psychological Benefits: Diabetes management involves lifestyle changes and ongoing vigilance, which can lead to stress and anxiety. The Mediterranean diet's rich array of flavorful, nutritious foods can enhance overall well-being and contribute to a positive relationship with food.

- Long-Term Health and Disease Prevention: Following the Mediterranean diet is not only beneficial for managing type 2 diabetes but can also contribute to overall health and well-being. Studies have shown that adhering to the Mediterranean diet is associated with a reduced risk of other chronic conditions such as certain cancers, Alzheimer's disease, and stroke.

2.1 Foods to Embrace

The Mediterranean diet emphasizes a wide array of wholesome, nutrient-rich foods, making it a flexible and enjoyable eating pattern. Some key foods to embrace include:

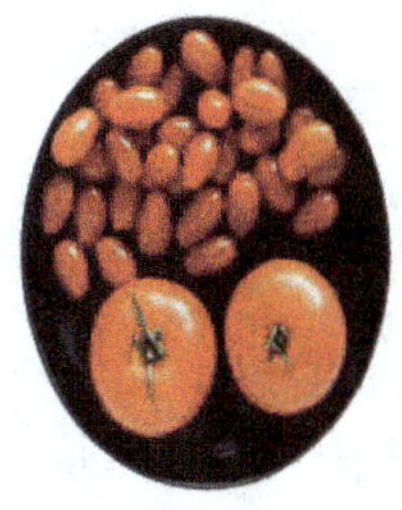

1.   Fruits and Vegetables: These form the foundation of the Mediterranean diet. Fresh, seasonal produce is abundant and provides essential vitamins, minerals, fiber, and antioxidants. Tomatoes, peppers, eggplants, leafy greens, berries, and citrus fruits are popular choices.

2.   Whole Grains: Whole grains such as whole wheat, oats, barley, quinoa, and brown rice are rich in fiber and essential nutrients. They provide sustained energy and help regulate blood sugar levels.

3. Healthy Fats: Olive oil is a staple in the Mediterranean diet and serves as the primary source of fat for cooking and dressing salads. Nuts, seeds, and avocados are also encouraged, providing a healthy dose of monounsaturated and polyunsaturated fats.

4. Legumes: Beans, lentils, chickpeas, and peas are excellent sources of plant-based protein, fiber, and minerals. They are versatile and can be included in soups, stews, salads, or as a side dish

5. Fish and Seafood: Fatty fish, such as salmon, sardines, mackerel, and trout, are rich in omega-3 fatty acids, which are essential for heart health and brain function. Regular consumption of fish provides valuable nutrients and may help reduce the risk of cardiovascular diseases.

6. Poultry: While red meat is limited, poultry like chicken and turkey can be included in moderate amounts as a source of lean protein.

7. Dairy: In the Mediterranean diet, dairy products like Greek yogurt and cheese are enjoyed in moderation, providing calcium and probiotics.

8. Herbs and Spices: Herbs and spices add depth and flavor to dishes, reducing the need for excess salt and enhancing the overall dining experience.

9. Water: Staying hydrated with water is fundamental to the Mediterranean lifestyle. Water is the primary beverage, and it is essential to limit sugary drinks and excessive alcohol consumption.

2.2 Foods to Limit or Avoid

While the Mediterranean diet celebrates a wide range of delicious and nutritious foods, there are certain items that should be limited or avoided to maintain the diet's health benefits:

- Red Meat and Processed Meats: Red meat, especially processed meats like sausages and bacon, should be consumed sparingly due to their association with an increased risk of heart disease and certain cancers.

- Sweets and Sugary Desserts: While the Mediterranean diet does not entirely eliminate sweets, these treats should be enjoyed in moderation and reserved for special occasions. Refined sugars and excessive consumption of desserts can lead to weight gain and negatively impact overall health.

- Highly Processed Foods: Processed foods that are high in refined sugars, unhealthy fats, and additives should be minimized. These foods often lack essential nutrients and may contribute to various health issues.

- Sodas and Sugary Beverages: Regular consumption of sugary sodas and beverages can lead to weight gain, insulin resistance, and an increased risk of type 2 diabetes. Water should be the primary beverage of choice.

- Excessive Alcohol: While moderate consumption of red wine has been associated with potential health benefits, excessive alcohol intake can have detrimental effects on health, including liver damage and increased risk of accidents.

- High-Sodium Foods: Processed and packaged foods, as well as excessive salt in cooking, should be limited. High sodium intake can contribute to hypertension and increase the risk of heart disease.

3.1 Mediterranean Diet and Type 2 Diabetes: Scientific Evidence

Over the past few decades, numerous research studies have explored the potential benefits of the Mediterranean diet in managing type 2 diabetes. These scientific investigations have consistently shown positive outcomes, supporting the idea that adopting a Mediterranean-style eating pattern can be an effective approach for individuals with type 2 diabetes.

A study published in the New England Journal of Medicine in 2013, known as the PREDIMED trial, demonstrated that participants who followed a Mediterranean diet supplemented with extra-virgin olive oil or mixed nuts had a significantly reduced risk of developing cardiovascular disease, which is a common complication associated with diabetes.

Another study published in the Annals of Internal Medicine in 2014 found that the Mediterranean diet was more effective at promoting weight loss and improving glycemic control compared to a low-fat diet, making it particularly beneficial for individuals with type 2 diabetes who struggle with obesity.

Numerous systematic reviews and meta-analyses have also confirmed the positive impact of the Mediterranean diet on various aspects of diabetes management, including blood sugar control, insulin sensitivity, and lipid profiles.

3.2 How the Diet Helps Manage Blood Sugar Levels

The Mediterranean diet's components work synergistically to help manage blood sugar levels and improve insulin sensitivity, making it a valuable tool for individuals with type 2 diabetes.

1. High Fiber Content: Fruits, vegetables, legumes, and whole grains are rich in dietary fiber. Fiber slows down the absorption of glucose in the bloodstream, preventing rapid spikes in blood sugar levels after meals.

2. Healthy Fats: The abundant use of olive oil, nuts, and fatty fish in the Mediterranean diet provides a steady source of healthy fats. These fats have been shown to improve insulin sensitivity and

reduce inflammation, which can contribute to better blood sugar regulation.

3. Low Glycemic Index: The Mediterranean diet emphasizes foods with a low glycemic index (GI), meaning they have a slower impact on blood sugar levels. Low-GI foods prevent sudden spikes and crashes in blood glucose, leading to more stable energy levels and reduced risk of diabetic complications.

4. Antioxidants and Anti-Inflammatory Properties: The diet's emphasis on fruits, vegetables, and herbs provides a rich source of antioxidants and anti-inflammatory compounds. Chronic inflammation is associated with insulin resistance and diabetes progression, and the antioxidants in the Mediterranean diet can help combat this inflammation.

5. Weight Management: The Mediterranean diet's focus on nutrient-dense, filling foods can aid in weight management, a crucial factor for

individuals with type 2 diabetes. Maintaining a healthy weight can improve insulin sensitivity and reduce the risk of cardiovascular complications.

6. Potential Gut Microbiota Benefits: Emerging research suggests that the Mediterranean diet's emphasis on plant-based foods may positively influence gut microbiota, the trillions of microorganisms living in the digestive tract. A healthy gut microbiome has been linked to better metabolic health, including improved blood sugar control.

3.3 Long-term Health Benefits and Potential for Diabetes Reversal

Beyond immediate blood sugar management, the Mediterranean diet offers a range of long-term health benefits that can positively impact individuals with type 2 diabetes. These benefits include:

- Cardiovascular Health: The Mediterranean diet's focus on heart-healthy fats, fiber, and antioxidants can reduce the risk of cardiovascular diseases, which are more prevalent in individuals with diabetes.

- Reduced Risk of Diabetes Complications: Following the Mediterranean diet can help lower the risk of diabetic complications such as nerve damage, kidney disease, and eye problems. The diet's nutrient-rich foods support overall health and can improve blood circulation and organ function.

- Sustainable Lifestyle: Unlike restrictive fad diets, the Mediterranean diet is a sustainable lifestyle approach that can be easily adopted and maintained for the long term. Its flexibility and variety make it enjoyable, increasing the likelihood of adhering to the diet over time.

- Diabetes Reversal Potential: Some research suggests that adopting a Mediterranean-style eating pattern, combined with regular physical activity and weight management, may lead to diabetes remission in some individuals. Reversal or remission of diabetes occurs when blood sugar levels return to normal without the need for medication. While not everyone may experience diabetes reversal, the Mediterranean diet can significantly improve diabetes management and reduce the reliance on medications for many individuals.

- Weight Management: Obesity and excess body weight are significant risk factors for type 2 diabetes. The Mediterranean diet's emphasis on whole, nutrient-dense foods can support healthy weight loss or maintenance, aiding in the prevention and management of diabetes

- Improved Quality of Life: Adopting the Mediterranean diet can lead to an overall improvement in the quality of life for individuals with type 2 diabetes. Better blood sugar control, increased energy levels, and a reduced risk of complications can enhance physical and mental well-being.

- Enhanced Insulin Sensitivity: Insulin resistance is a core issue in type 2 diabetes, where the body's cells become less responsive to insulin's effects. The Mediterranean diet has been shown to improve insulin sensitivity, allowing the body to use insulin more effectively and regulate blood sugar levels more efficiently.

- Reduced Inflammation: Chronic inflammation is associated with various chronic diseases, including type 2 diabetes. The Mediterranean diet's anti-inflammatory properties, derived from its abundant antioxidant-rich foods, can help combat inflammation and potentially slow down disease progression.

- Lowered Risk of Metabolic Syndrome: Metabolic syndrome is a cluster of conditions, including high blood pressure, high blood sugar, excess body fat, and abnormal cholesterol levels. The Mediterranean diet has been associated with a reduced risk of metabolic syndrome, which is closely linked to the development of type 2 diabetes.

- Prevention of Type 2 Diabetes: Even in individuals without diabetes, adopting the Mediterranean diet can be a preventive measure against developing type 2 diabetes. Its focus on healthy eating and lifestyle habits can reduce the risk factors associated with the onset of the disease.

- Enhanced Heart Health: The Mediterranean diet's impact on heart health is not only beneficial for individuals with diabetes but for the general population as well. It can help lower LDL cholesterol levels, reduce blood pressure, and decrease the risk of heart disease, which is a significant concern for those with diabetes.

- Potential for Positive Mental Health: Although not directly related to blood sugar management, the Mediterranean diet's emphasis on nutrient-dense foods and omega-3 fatty acids has been associated with improved mood and mental well-being. Managing diabetes can be emotionally challenging, and the diet's psychological benefits can be invaluable.

Part 1: Breakfast Delights

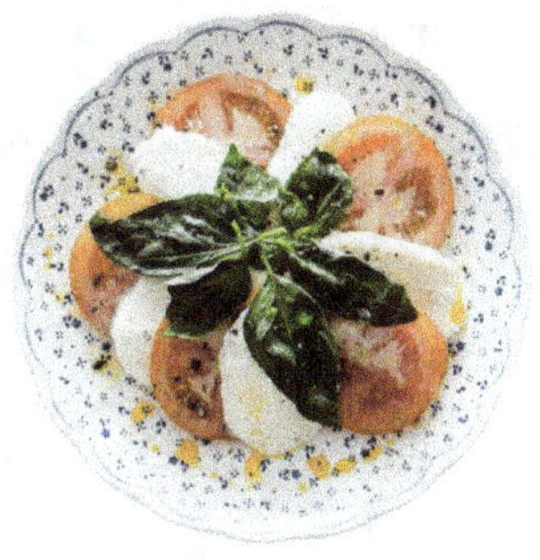

5.1 Greek Yogurt Parfait with Fresh Fruits and Nuts

Ingredients

- 1 cup Greek yogurt (unsweetened and low-fat)

- 1/2 cup mixed fresh fruits (e.g., berries, sliced peaches, or pomegranate seeds)

- 2 tablespoons chopped nuts (e.g., almonds, walnuts, or pistachios)

- 1 teaspoon honey (optional, for added sweetness)

- 1/2 teaspoon vanilla extract

- A pinch of cinnamon (optional, for added flavor)

Step by Step Preparation

1. In a small bowl, mix the Greek yogurt, vanilla extract, and cinnamon (if using). The vanilla extract adds a delightful aroma and flavor, while the cinnamon provides additional sweetness without the need for excess sugar.

2. Layer the Greek yogurt mixture with the fresh fruits in a glass or a parfait dish. Start with a dollop of yogurt at the bottom of the glass, followed by a layer of mixed fruits, and then repeat the process until the glass is filled.

3. Top the parfait with chopped nuts. Nuts not only add crunch and flavor but also provide healthy fats, which can help slow down the absorption of sugar and contribute to better blood sugar control.

4. If you prefer a sweeter taste, drizzle a teaspoon of honey over the top. However, it's essential to use

honey in moderation, as it contains natural sugars.

5. Serve the Greek Yogurt Parfait immediately or refrigerate for a short time to allow the flavors to meld.

Variations:

- Seeds: Instead of nuts, you can sprinkle chia seeds or flax seeds on top of the parfait for an extra boost of fiber and omega-3 fatty acids.

- Mint Leaves: Garnish with fresh mint leaves for a refreshing touch.

- Granola: If you enjoy a bit of crunch, you can add a small amount of low-sugar granola between the layers.

- Other Fruits: Get creative and use your favorite seasonal fruits or mix different fruits to add variety to your parfait.

5.2 Turkish Shakshuka with Spinach and Feta

Ingredients

- 2 tablespoons olive oil

- 1 small onion, finely chopped

- 2 cloves garlic, minced

- 1 red bell pepper, diced

- 1 yellow bell pepper, diced

- 1 teaspoon ground cumin

- 1 teaspoon ground paprika

- 1/2 teaspoon ground cayenne pepper (adjust to your spice preference)

- 1 can (14 ounces) diced tomatoes (no added sugar)

- 2 cups fresh spinach, chopped

- 4-6 large eggs (depending on the number of servings)

- 1/2 cup crumbled feta cheese

- Salt and pepper to taste

- Fresh parsley, chopped (for garnish)

Step by Step Preparation

1. In a large skillet or a shallow pan, heat the olive oil over medium heat.

2. Add the chopped onion and sauté until it becomes translucent, about 2-3 minutes.

3. Stir in the minced garlic and cook for an additional minute until the garlic becomes fragrant.

4. Add the diced red and yellow bell peppers to the pan and cook for 3-4 minutes until they start to soften.

5. Sprinkle the ground cumin, paprika, and cayenne pepper over the vegetables. Stir well to coat the vegetables with the spices.

6. Pour the canned diced tomatoes (with their juice) into the pan. Season with salt and pepper to taste. Simmer the sauce for about 5-7 minutes, allowing the flavors to meld and the sauce to thicken slightly.

7. Add the chopped spinach to the tomato sauce and gently stir until the spinach wilts down.

8. Create small wells in the sauce and carefully crack the eggs into each well. Cover the pan with a lid and let the eggs poach for 5-7 minutes or until the egg whites are set, but the yolks are still runny. If you prefer well-cooked eggs, you can cook them a bit longer.

9. Sprinkle the crumbled feta cheese over the top of the shakshuka.

10. Garnish with chopped fresh parsley for a burst of color and added flavor.

11. Serve the Turkish Shakshuka with crusty whole-grain bread or pita on the side for a complete and satisfying meal.

Variations:

- Veggies: Feel free to add other vegetables such as zucchini, mushrooms, or eggplant to the shakshuka to increase the nutritional value and add variety.

- Spices: Adjust the spice levels to your preference. If you prefer a milder flavor, reduce the amount of cayenne pepper.

- Cheese: If you're not a fan of feta cheese, you can substitute it with another Mediterranean cheese like goat cheese or use a low-fat mozzarella.

- Egg Substitute: If you want to make this dish vegan-friendly, you can use tofu or a plant-based egg substitute in place of the eggs.

5.3 Italian Frittata with Sun-Dried Tomatoes and Basil

Ingredients

- 6 large eggs

- 1/4 cup milk (you can use low-fat or plant-based milk)

- 1/4 cup grated Parmesan cheese (optional, for added flavor)

- 1/4 cup sun-dried tomatoes, chopped (ensure they are not packed in oil)

- 1/4 cup fresh basil leaves, chopped

- 1 small onion, finely chopped

- 2 cloves garlic, minced

- 1 tablespoon olive oil

- Salt and pepper to taste

Step by Step Preparation

1. Preheat your oven's broiler.

2. In a medium-sized bowl, whisk the eggs, milk, grated Parmesan (if using), salt, and pepper until well combined. The milk adds moisture and helps create a fluffy texture.

3. In an oven-safe skillet (preferably non-stick), heat the olive oil over medium heat.

4. Add the chopped onion and sauté until it becomes translucent, about 2-3 minutes.

5. Stir in the minced garlic and cook for an additional minute until the garlic becomes fragrant.

6. Add the chopped sun-dried tomatoes to the skillet and cook for another 2 minutes to allow the flavors to meld.

7. Pour the egg mixture over the sautéed vegetables in the skillet.

8. Reduce the heat to low and let the frittata cook gently for about 5 minutes until the edges are set, but the center is still slightly runny.

9. Sprinkle the chopped basil leaves over the top of the frittata.

10. Place the skillet under the broiler for about 2-3 minutes or until the top of the frittata is golden brown and fully set.

11. Remove the skillet from the oven (careful, it will be hot!) and let the frittata cool for a minute or two.

12. Use a spatula to carefully slide the frittata onto a serving plate.

13. Slice the frittata into wedges and serve warm.

<u>*Variations*</u>:

- Vegetables: Feel free to add other vegetables such as bell peppers, zucchini, or spinach to the frittata for added nutrients and flavor.

- Cheese: If you prefer a creamier frittata, you can add some crumbled goat cheese or feta cheese to the egg mixture.

- Herbs: Aside from basil, you can experiment with other fresh herbs like parsley, oregano, or thyme, depending on your taste preference.

- Meat Option: If you want to add a protein boost, you can include cooked and crumbled turkey sausage or lean ham in the frittata.

PART 2: Wholesome Lunches

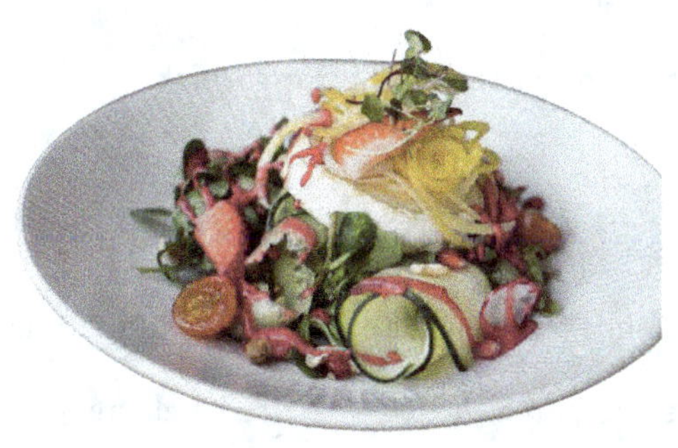

6.1 Spanish Gazpacho with Avocado and Cucumber

Ingredients

- 4 large ripe tomatoes, chopped

- 1 cucumber, peeled and chopped

- 1 red bell pepper, chopped

- 1 small red onion, chopped

- 2 cloves garlic, minced

- 1 avocado, peeled and diced

- 2 cups tomato juice (no added sugar)

- 2 tablespoons red wine vinegar

- 2 tablespoons extra-virgin olive oil

- 1/2 teaspoon ground cumin

- Salt and pepper to taste

- Fresh basil or parsley leaves for garnish

Step by Step Preparation

1. In a blender or food processor, combine the chopped tomatoes, cucumber, red bell pepper, red onion, and minced garlic. Blend until the vegetables are finely pureed.

2. Add the avocado to the blender and blend again until the mixture becomes smooth and creamy.

3. Pour the tomato juice, red wine vinegar, and extra-virgin olive oil into the blender. Sprinkle in the ground cumin, salt, and pepper to taste. Blend the ingredients until everything is well combined.

4. Taste the Gazpacho and adjust the seasonings according to your preference. You can add more salt, pepper, or vinegar as needed.

5. Transfer the Gazpacho to a large bowl or container and refrigerate it for at least 1-2 hours to chill and allow the flavors to meld.

6. Before serving, give the Gazpacho a good stir. If it has thickened too much, you can add a splash of tomato juice to reach your desired consistency.

7. Garnish the Gazpacho with fresh basil or parsley leaves for a pop of color and added freshness.

8. Serve the Spanish Gazpacho with Avocado and Cucumber in chilled bowls or glasses for a cooling and nutritious treat.

<u>*Variations*</u>:

- Spice it up: If you prefer a spicier version, you can add a dash of hot sauce or a sprinkle of cayenne pepper to the Gazpacho.

- Texture: If you like a chunkier Gazpacho, you can reserve some chopped vegetables and avocado to stir in just before serving.

- Herbs: Experiment with different fresh herbs like cilantro or dill to add unique flavors to the Gazpacho.

- Croutons: For added texture and a bit of crunch, top the Gazpacho with homemade whole-grain croutons.

6.2 Moroccan Chickpea Salad with Roasted Vegetables

Ingredients

<u>*For the Salad*</u>:

- 1 can (15 ounces) chickpeas, drained and rinsed

- 1 red bell pepper, chopped

- 1 yellow bell pepper, chopped

- 1 zucchini, chopped

- 1 red onion, sliced

- 2 tablespoons olive oil

- 1 teaspoon ground cumin

- 1 teaspoon ground coriander

- 1/2 teaspoon ground cinnamon

- Salt and pepper to taste

- 1/4 cup chopped fresh parsley or cilantro (for garnish)

For the Dressing:

- 3 tablespoons extra-virgin olive oil

- 2 tablespoons lemon juice

- 1 clove garlic, minced

- 1/2 teaspoon ground cumin

- 1/2 teaspoon ground coriander

- Salt and pepper to taste

Step by Step Preparation

1. Preheat your oven to 400°F (200°C).

2. In a large mixing bowl, combine the chopped red and yellow bell peppers, zucchini, and sliced red onion.

3. In a small bowl, mix together the olive oil, ground cumin, ground coriander, ground cinnamon, salt, and pepper to create the spice blend.

4. Drizzle the spice blend over the chopped vegetables and toss until the vegetables are evenly coated.

5. Spread the seasoned vegetables in a single layer on a baking sheet lined with parchment paper or a silicone baking mat.

6. Roast the vegetables in the preheated oven for about 25-30 minutes or until they are tender and slightly caramelized, stirring them halfway through the cooking time.

7. While the vegetables are roasting, prepare the dressing by whisking together the extra-virgin olive oil, lemon juice, minced garlic, ground cumin, ground coriander, salt, and pepper in a small bowl.

8. In a large salad bowl, combine the roasted vegetables and the drained and rinsed chickpeas.

9. Pour the dressing over the chickpeas and roasted vegetables. Toss everything together until the salad is well coated with the dressing.

10. Garnish the Moroccan Chickpea Salad with Roasted Vegetables with chopped fresh parsley or cilantro.

11. Serve the salad at room temperature or refrigerate for a while to let the flavors meld before serving.

Variations:

- Spices: Feel free to adjust the spices according to your taste preference. You can add a pinch of cayenne pepper for a bit of heat.

- Vegetables: You can add other roasted vegetables such as eggplant, carrots, or sweet potatoes to the salad for added variety and nutrients.

- Nuts: To add some crunch and healthy fats, you can sprinkle toasted almonds or pine nuts on top of the salad.

- Greens: For an extra boost of freshness, you can serve the salad on a bed of baby spinach or arugula.

6.3 Lebanese Lentil Soup with Spinach and Lemon

Ingredients

- 1 cup dried red lentils, rinsed and drained

- 1 large onion, finely chopped

- 3 cloves garlic, minced

- 1 tablespoon olive oil

- 1 teaspoon ground cumin

- 1/2 teaspoon ground coriander

- 1/2 teaspoon ground turmeric

- 1/4 teaspoon ground cinnamon

- 6 cups low-sodium vegetable broth

- 4 cups fresh spinach leaves, roughly chopped

- Zest and juice of 1 lemon

- Salt and pepper to taste

- Fresh parsley or cilantro, chopped, for garnish

Step by Step Preparation

1. In a large soup pot or Dutch oven, heat the olive oil over medium heat.

2. Add the chopped onion and sauté until it becomes translucent, about 2-3 minutes.

3. Stir in the minced garlic and cook for an additional minute until the garlic becomes fragrant.

4. Add the ground cumin, ground coriander, ground turmeric, and ground cinnamon to the pot. Stir

the spices with the onions and garlic to release their flavors.

5. Add the rinsed lentils to the pot and toss them with the spices and aromatics.

6. Pour in the vegetable broth and bring the mixture to a boil.

7. Once it reaches a boil, reduce the heat to low, cover the pot, and let the soup simmer for about 20-25 minutes or until the lentils become tender.

8. Stir in the chopped spinach leaves and let them wilt in the hot soup.

9. Add the lemon zest and lemon juice to the soup, and season with salt and pepper to taste. The lemon adds a bright, citrusy flavor that compliments the earthy lentils.

10. Give the soup a taste and adjust the seasonings, adding more lemon juice or spices if desired.

11. Ladle the Lebanese Lentil Soup into bowls and garnish with chopped fresh parsley or cilantro.

12. Serve the soup hot and enjoy the comforting flavors of this Mediterranean-inspired dish.

<u>*Variations*</u>:

- Herbs: For an extra burst of freshness, you can add a tablespoon of chopped fresh mint or a few dashes of dried mint to the soup.

- Vegetables: Feel free to add other vegetables like carrots or diced tomatoes to the soup for added texture and nutrients.

- Creamy Texture: If you prefer a creamier soup, you can use an immersion blender to partially blend the soup, creating a thicker consistency.

- Spice Level: Adjust the amount of spices to suit your taste preferences. You can add more or less ground cumin, coriander, or cinnamon to your liking.

PART 3: Nourishing Dinners

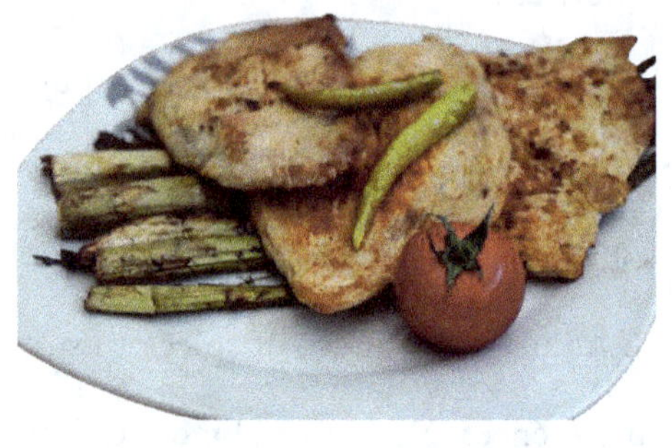

7.1 Greek Grilled Fish with Herbs and Lemon

Ingredients

- 4 fish filets (such as sea bass, trout, or snapper), about 4-6 ounces each

- 2 tablespoons extra-virgin olive oil

- 2 tablespoons fresh lemon juice

- 2 cloves garlic, minced

- 1 tablespoon fresh oregano, chopped (or 1 teaspoon dried oregano)

- 1 tablespoon fresh parsley, chopped

- 1 tablespoon fresh thyme leaves (or 1 teaspoon dried thyme)

- 1 teaspoon fresh rosemary, chopped (or 1/2 teaspoon dried rosemary)

- Zest of 1 lemon

- Salt and pepper to taste

- Lemon wedges, for serving

Step by Step Preparation

1. In a small bowl, whisk together the olive oil, lemon juice, minced garlic, chopped oregano,

parsley, thyme, rosemary, and lemon zest to create the marinade.

2. Place the fish filets in a shallow dish or a large resealable plastic bag.

3. Pour the marinade over the fish, ensuring that all sides are coated. Cover the dish or seal the bag and refrigerate for at least 30 minutes to allow the flavors to infuse.

4. Preheat the grill to medium-high heat. Make sure to lightly oil the grates to prevent sticking.

5. Remove the fish from the marinade and let any excess marinade drip off.

6. Season the fish with salt and pepper to taste.

7. Grill the fish filets for about 4-5 minutes on each side, or until the fish is cooked through and flakes easily with a fork. Cooking time may vary depending on the thickness of the filets.

8. Once the fish is grilled to perfection, remove it from the grill and let it rest for a minute before serving.

9. Garnish the Greek Grilled Fish with extra fresh herbs and lemon wedges for an added burst of flavor.

10. Serve the fish with a side of Mediterranean-inspired vegetables or a fresh salad for a complete and nutritious meal.

Variations:

- Herb Choices: If you prefer different herbs, you can customize the recipe with your favorites, such as basil, dill, or mint.

- Lemon Garlic Butter: For a richer flavor, you can melt some garlic-infused butter and drizzle it over the grilled fish before serving.

- Grill or Oven: If you don't have a grill, you can also cook the fish in the oven. Preheat the oven to 400°F (200°C) and bake the fish for about 10-15 minutes, or until cooked through.

- Fish Choices: Feel free to use your preferred fish filets, making sure they are fresh and sustainably sourced.

7.2 Italian Ratatouille with Olives and Capers

Ingredients

- 1 eggplant, diced into 1-inch cubes
- 1 zucchini, diced into 1-inch cubes
- 1 yellow bell pepper, diced
- 1 red bell pepper, diced
- 1 large onion, chopped
- 3 cloves garlic, minced
- 2 tablespoons extra-virgin olive oil
- 1 can (14 ounces) diced tomatoes (preferably fire-roasted)
- 1 tablespoon tomato paste
- 1 teaspoon dried oregano
- 1 teaspoon dried basil
- 1/2 teaspoon dried thyme

- 1/4 teaspoon red pepper flakes (optional, for a bit of heat)

- Salt and pepper to taste

- 1/4 cup pitted Kalamata olives, halved

- 2 tablespoons capers, drained

- Fresh basil leaves, for garnish

Step by Step Preparation

1. Preheat the oven to 400°F (200°C).

2. In a large oven-safe skillet or a Dutch oven, heat the olive oil over medium heat.

3. Add the chopped onion to the skillet and sauté until it becomes translucent, about 2-3 minutes.

4. Stir in the minced garlic and cook for an additional minute until the garlic becomes fragrant.

5. Add the diced eggplant, zucchini, yellow bell pepper, and red bell pepper to the skillet. Season with salt and pepper to taste.

6. Sauté the vegetables for about 5 minutes until they begin to soften.

7. Stir in the diced tomatoes, tomato paste, dried oregano, dried basil, dried thyme, and red pepper flakes (if using). Mix well to combine all the flavors.

8. Let the ratatouille simmer on the stovetop for about 5 minutes to allow the flavors to meld.

9. Once the mixture is heated through, transfer the skillet to the preheated oven.

10. Roast the ratatouille in the oven for about 20-25 minutes or until the vegetables are tender and slightly caramelized.

11. Remove the skillet from the oven and stir in the halved Kalamata olives and drained capers.

12. Garnish the Italian Ratatouille with fresh basil leaves for an extra touch of flavor and aroma.

13. Serve the ratatouille warm as a main dish or a side, and enjoy the hearty and wholesome flavors of this Mediterranean-inspired delight.

<u>Variations</u>:

- Herbs: If you have fresh herbs on hand, feel free to use them instead of dried herbs for an even more robust flavor.

- Vegetables: You can add other vegetables like tomatoes, mushrooms, or artichoke hearts to the ratatouille for added variety.

- Protein: For a complete meal, you can add some cooked chickpeas, cannellini beans, or grilled chicken to the ratatouille.

- Cheese: If you'd like, you can sprinkle some crumbled feta or grated Parmesan cheese on top before serving.

7.3 Turkish Baked Eggplant with Ground Lamb and Spices

Ingredients

- 2 large eggplants

- 1/2 lb (225g) lean ground lamb (you can also use lean ground beef or turkey)

- 1 large onion, finely chopped

- 3 cloves garlic, minced

- 1 tablespoon olive oil

- 1 can (14 ounces) diced tomatoes (preferably fire-roasted)

- 2 tablespoons tomato paste

- 1 teaspoon ground cumin

- 1 teaspoon ground coriander

- 1/2 teaspoon ground cinnamon

- 1/4 teaspoon ground allspice

- Pinch of cayenne pepper (optional, for heat)

- Salt and pepper to taste

- Fresh parsley, chopped, for garnish

- Greek yogurt, for serving (optional)

Step by Step Preparation

1. Preheat the oven to 400°F (200°C).

2. Wash the eggplants and trim off the stems. Cut the eggplants in half lengthwise.

3. Use a sharp knife to score the flesh of each eggplant half in a criss-cross pattern. Be careful not to cut through the skin.

4. Sprinkle some salt over the scored eggplant halves and let them sit for about 15 minutes. This step helps to remove excess moisture and bitterness from the eggplants.

5. While the eggplants are resting, prepare the filling. In a large skillet, heat the olive oil over medium heat.

6. Add the chopped onion to the skillet and sauté until it becomes translucent, about 2-3 minutes.

7. Stir in the minced garlic and cook for an additional minute until the garlic becomes fragrant.

8. Add the ground lamb to the skillet and cook until it browns and is no longer pink.

9. Stir in the diced tomatoes, tomato paste, ground cumin, ground coriander, ground cinnamon, ground allspice, and cayenne pepper (if using). Season with salt and pepper to taste. Mix well to combine all the flavors.

10. Let the filling simmer for about 5-7 minutes, allowing the flavors to meld together.

11. While the filling is simmering, rinse the eggplant halves under cold water and pat them dry with a paper towel.

12. Place the eggplant halves on a baking sheet, scored side up.

13. Fill each eggplant half generously with the lamb and tomato mixture, pressing it into the scorched flesh.

14. Bake the Turkish Baked Eggplant in the preheated oven for about 25-30 minutes, or until the eggplants are tender and slightly caramelized.

15. Remove the baking sheet from the oven and garnish the eggplants with freshly chopped parsley.

16. Serve the Turkish Baked Eggplant with a dollop of Greek yogurt on the side (optional) for a creamy and cooling contrast to the savory flavors.

Variations:

- Spices: Feel free to adjust the spices according to your taste preferences. You can add more or less cumin, coriander, cinnamon, or allspice to suit your liking.

- Vegetarian Option: For a meatless version, you can substitute the ground lamb with cooked lentils or chickpeas.

- Cheese: If you enjoy cheese, you can sprinkle some crumbled feta or grated Parmesan on top before serving.

PART 4: Sides and Snacks

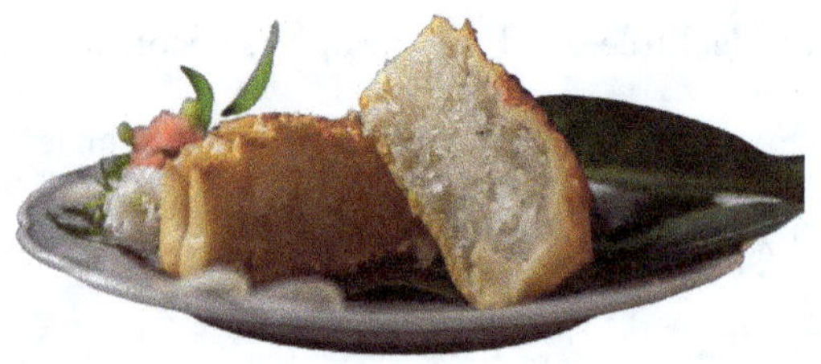

8.1 Spanish Stuffed Bell Peppers with Quinoa and Herbs

Ingredients

- 4 large bell peppers (red, yellow, or orange), tops removed and seeds removed

- 1 cup cooked quinoa (prepared according to package instructions)

- 1 can (14 ounces) diced tomatoes (preferably fire-roasted)

- 1 cup cooked black beans (canned or homemade)

- 1/2 cup chopped cherry tomatoes

- 1/2 cup chopped cucumber

- 1/4 cup chopped red onion

- 1/4 cup chopped fresh parsley

- 2 tablespoons chopped fresh mint

- 2 tablespoons chopped fresh basil

- 1 tablespoon extra-virgin olive oil

- 2 cloves garlic, minced

- 1 teaspoon ground cumin

- 1/2 teaspoon smoked paprika

- Salt and pepper to taste

- Crumbled feta cheese, for garnish (optional)

Step by Step Preparation

1. Preheat the oven to 375°F (190°C).

2. In a large pot, bring water to a boil and cook the quinoa according to the package instructions. Once cooked, set aside.

3. In a skillet, heat the olive oil over medium heat.

4. Add the minced garlic, ground cumin, and smoked paprika to the skillet. Sauté for about 1 minute until the spices become fragrant.

5. Stir in the diced tomatoes and cooked black beans. Cook for another 2-3 minutes, allowing the flavors to blend.

6. Remove the skillet from the heat and transfer the mixture to a large mixing bowl.

7. To the bowl, add the cooked quinoa, chopped cherry tomatoes, cucumber, red onion, parsley, mint, and basil.

8. Mix all the ingredients together until well combined. Season with salt and pepper to taste.

9. Prepare the bell peppers by cutting off the tops and removing the seeds and membranes.

10. Stuff each bell pepper with the quinoa and herb mixture, pressing it down gently to ensure the peppers are filled evenly.

11. Place the stuffed bell peppers in a baking dish.

12. Cover the dish with aluminum foil and bake in the preheated oven for about 25-30 minutes, or until the bell peppers are tender.

13. Remove the foil and bake for an additional 5-7 minutes to slightly brown the tops.

14. Once the Spanish Stuffed Bell Peppers are ready, garnish with crumbled feta cheese (if using) and an extra sprinkle of fresh herbs.

15. Serve the stuffed bell peppers hot and savor the vibrant flavors of this Mediterranean-inspired dish.

Variations:

- Vegetables: Feel free to add other vegetables such as chopped spinach, artichoke hearts, or roasted red peppers to the quinoa stuffing.

- Protein: For a different protein source, you can use cooked ground turkey or chicken instead of black beans.

- Nuts: For added texture and healthy fats, you can mix in some chopped almonds, walnuts, or pine nuts.

- Spice Level: Adjust the spices to your liking by adding more or less cumin and smoked paprika, or adding a dash of chili powder for extra heat.

8.2 Moroccan Hummus with Tahini and Cumin

Ingredients

- 1 can (15 ounces) chickpeas, drained and rinsed

- 1/4 cup tahini

- 2 tablespoons fresh lemon juice

- 2 cloves garlic, minced

- 1 teaspoon ground cumin

- 1/2 teaspoon ground paprika

- 1/4 teaspoon ground cinnamon

- 2 tablespoons extra-virgin olive oil

- Salt to taste

- Fresh parsley, chopped, for garnish

- Extra olive oil, for drizzling

- Whole wheat pita bread or vegetable sticks, for serving

Step by Step Preparation

1. In a food processor, combine the chickpeas, tahini, lemon juice, minced garlic, ground cumin, ground paprika, and ground cinnamon.

2. Process the ingredients until they are well blended and start to form a smooth paste.

3. While the food processor is running, gradually add the olive oil in a steady stream until the hummus reaches your desired consistency. If

needed, add a tablespoon or two of water to thin it out.

4. Taste the hummus and season with salt according to your preference. Adjust the flavors by adding more lemon juice, garlic, or spices if desired.

5. Transfer the Moroccan Hummus to a serving bowl.

6. Drizzle some extra olive oil over the top and garnish with freshly chopped parsley.

7. Serve the hummus with whole wheat pita bread or a selection of vegetable sticks such as carrot, cucumber, and bell pepper.

__Variations__:

- Spice Level: If you prefer a spicier hummus, you can add a pinch of cayenne pepper or a dash of hot sauce to the mixture.

- Roasted Vegetables: For added flavor and texture, you can top the hummus with roasted vegetables such as diced eggplant, bell peppers, or cherry tomatoes.

- Herbs: Experiment with different herbs such as fresh cilantro, mint, or basil to add a unique twist to your hummus.

- Nuts and Seeds: For added crunch and nutritional value, you can sprinkle some toasted sesame seeds, chopped almonds, or pine nuts on top of the hummus.

8.3 Lebanese Tabbouleh with Fresh Parsley and Mint

Ingredients

- 1 cup bulgur wheat

- 2 cups boiling water

- 1 large bunch fresh parsley, finely chopped

- 1/2 cup fresh mint leaves, finely chopped

- 1 cup cherry tomatoes, halved

- 1/2 cup cucumber, diced

- 1/4 cup red onion, finely chopped

- 1/4 cup extra-virgin olive oil

- 1/4 cup fresh lemon juice

- Salt and pepper to taste

- Lettuce leaves, for serving

- Lemon wedges, for garnish

Step by Step Preparation

1. Place the bulgur wheat in a large bowl and pour the boiling water over it. Cover the bowl with a lid or plate and let it sit for about 20-25 minutes, or until the bulgur is tender and has absorbed the water.

2. While the bulgur is soaking, prepare the vegetables. Wash and chop the fresh parsley, mint leaves, cherry tomatoes, cucumber, and red onion.

3. In a separate small bowl, whisk together the extra-virgin olive oil, fresh lemon juice, salt, and pepper to create the dressing.

4. Once the bulgur is ready, fluff it with a fork to separate the grains.

5. Add the chopped parsley, mint, cherry tomatoes, cucumber, and red onion to the bulgur. Mix well to combine all the ingredients.

6. Pour the dressing over the tabouleh salad and toss until everything is evenly coated.

7. Taste and adjust the seasoning, adding more salt, pepper, or lemon juice as needed.

8. To serve, arrange some lettuce leaves on a platter or individual plates.

9. Spoon the Lebanese Tabbouleh onto the lettuce leaves.

10. Garnish with lemon wedges and a few extra mint leaves for a fresh touch.

Variations:

- Quinoa Tabbouleh: For a gluten-free version, you can substitute the bulgur wheat with cooked quinoa.

- Additional Vegetables: Feel free to add other vegetables such as diced bell peppers, radishes, or even some chopped olives for added texture and flavor.

- Protein Boost: To turn this tabbouleh into a more substantial meal, you can add some cooked chickpeas or grilled chicken on top.

- Nuts and Seeds: For extra crunch and healthy fats, sprinkle some toasted pine nuts or slivered almonds over the tabouleh.

PART 5: Desserts and Treats

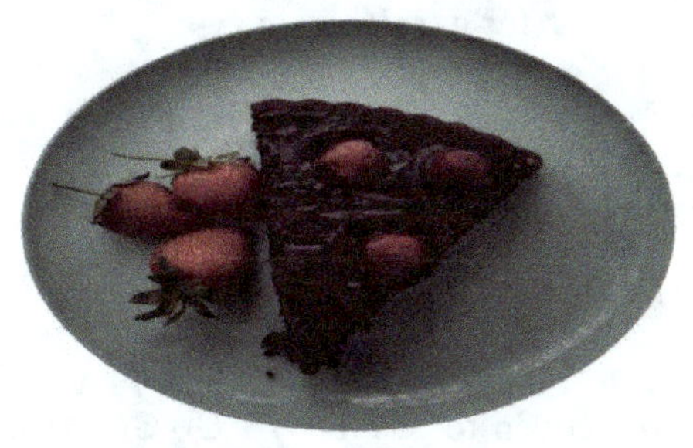

9.1 Greek Orange and Almond Cake

Ingredients

- 3 large oranges

- 4 eggs

- 1 cup almond flour

- 1 cup all-purpose flour (or whole wheat flour for a healthier option)

- 1 cup granulated sweetener (such as stevia or erythritol) or regular sugar

- 1 teaspoon baking powder

- 1/4 teaspoon salt

- 1/4 cup extra-virgin olive oil

- 1 teaspoon pure vanilla extract

- Sliced almonds, for garnish

- Powdered sweetener (optional), for dusting

Step by Step Preparation

1. Preheat your oven to 350°F (175°C). Grease a 9-inch round cake pan and line the bottom with parchment paper for easy removal.

2. Wash the oranges thoroughly. Place them in a saucepan and cover them with water. Bring the water to a boil, then reduce the heat to a simmer.

Cook the oranges for about 1 hour until they are tender. Drain and let them cool.

3. Once the oranges are cool, cut them into quarters and remove any seeds. Place the oranges (including the skin) into a food processor or blender. Pulse until you have a smooth puree.

4. In a large mixing bowl, beat the eggs and sweetener (or sugar) together until well combined.

5. Add the almond flour, all-purpose flour (or whole wheat flour), baking powder, and salt to the bowl. Mix everything together until you have a smooth batter.

6. Stir in the orange puree, extra-virgin olive oil, and vanilla extract. Continue mixing until all the ingredients are fully incorporated.

7. Pour the batter into the prepared cake pan and spread it evenly.

8. Sprinkle sliced almonds over the top of the cake for added texture and presentation.

9. Bake the cake in the preheated oven for approximately 40-45 minutes or until a toothpick inserted in the center comes out clean.

10. Once the cake is done, remove it from the oven and let it cool in the pan for about 10 minutes.

11. Carefully transfer the cake to a wire rack to cool completely.

12. If desired, dust the top of the cake with powdered sweetener before serving.

Variations:

- Gluten-Free Option: To make this cake gluten-free, use gluten-free all-purpose flour or a gluten-free baking mix instead of regular flour.

- Citrus Twist: Experiment with different citrus fruits such as lemons or blood oranges to create unique variations of this cake.

- Nut-Free Alternative: If you have nut allergies, you can use coconut flour or a gluten-free flour blend instead of almond flour.

- Yogurt Topping: Serve the cake with a dollop of Greek yogurt on the side for added creaminess and tang.

9.2 Italian Olive Oil and Rosemary Biscotti

Ingredients

- 2 cups all-purpose flour (or whole wheat flour for a healthier option)

- 1 teaspoon baking powder

- 1/4 teaspoon salt

- 1/2 cup granulated sweetener (such as stevia or erythritol) or regular sugar

- 1/4 cup extra-virgin olive oil

- 2 large eggs

- 1 tablespoon fresh rosemary, finely chopped

- Zest of 1 lemon

- 1 teaspoon pure vanilla extract

- 1/2 cup almonds, coarsely chopped

Step by Step Preparation

1. Preheat your oven to 350°F (175°C). Line a baking sheet with parchment paper.

2. In a medium-sized mixing bowl, whisk together the flour, baking powder, and salt.

3. In a separate large bowl, whisk together the sweetener (or sugar), extra-virgin olive oil, and eggs until well combined.

4. Stir in the chopped rosemary, lemon zest, and pure vanilla extract.

5. Gradually add the dry ingredients to the wet ingredients, mixing until a dough forms.

6. Fold in the coarsely chopped almonds, distributing them evenly throughout the dough.

7. On a floured surface, divide the dough into two equal portions.

8. Shape each portion into a log about 10 inches long and 2 inches wide, placing them on the prepared baking sheet, leaving space between them.

9. Bake the biscotti logs in the preheated oven for about 20-25 minutes or until they are lightly golden and firm to the touch.

10. Remove the biscotti logs from the oven and let them cool on the baking sheet for about 15 minutes.

11. Reduce the oven temperature to 325°F (160°C).

12. Once the biscotti logs have cooled slightly, transfer them to a cutting board and slice them diagonally into 1/2-inch thick pieces using a sharp knife.

13. Lay the biscotti slices flat on the baking sheet and return them to the oven.

14. Bake the biscotti slices for an additional 10-15 minutes, flipping them over halfway through to

ensure even baking. The biscotti should be crisp and lightly toasted.

15. Remove the biscotti from the oven and let them cool completely on a wire rack.

<u>*Variations*</u>:

- Citrus Twist: Instead of lemon zest, you can use orange zest for a slightly different citrus flavor.

- Nut-Free Option: If you have nut allergies, you can omit the almonds or replace them with dried cranberries or raisins for added sweetness and texture.

- Chocolate Drizzle: For an occasional indulgence, you can drizzle melted dark chocolate over the cooled biscotti.

- Herb Substitution: If you prefer a different herb flavor, you can use fresh thyme or even a pinch of ground cinnamon for a warm touch.

9.3 Turkish Baklava with Walnuts and Honey

Ingredients

- 1 package (16 ounces) of phyllo dough, thawed (keep it covered with a damp cloth to prevent drying)
- 1 1/2 cups walnuts, finely chopped
- 1/4 cup granulated sweetener (such as stevia or erythritol) or regular sugar
- 1 teaspoon ground cinnamon
- 1/2 cup unsalted butter, melted
- 1 cup honey
- 1/2 cup water
- 1 teaspoon fresh lemon juice

Step by Step Preparation

1. Preheat your oven to 350°F (175°C). Grease a 9x13-inch baking dish with a little melted butter.
2. In a bowl, mix the chopped walnuts, sweetener (or sugar), and ground cinnamon until well combined. Set the nut mixture aside.

3. Unroll the phyllo dough and place it on a clean, dry surface. Cover it with a damp cloth to prevent it from drying out while you work.

4. Carefully layer half of the phyllo sheets in the prepared baking dish, brushing each sheet with melted butter as you go. Make sure to cover the bottom completely.

5. Spread the walnut mixture evenly over the layered phyllo sheets.

6. Layer the remaining phyllo sheets on top of the nut mixture, brushing each sheet with butter again.

7. Using a sharp knife, cut the baklava into diamond or square shapes by making diagonal cuts. This will help the syrup to penetrate and flavor the dessert evenly.

8. Bake the baklava in the preheated oven for about 40-45 minutes or until it turns golden brown and crispy.

9.   While the baklava is baking, prepare the honey syrup. In a saucepan, combine the honey, water, and fresh lemon juice. Bring the mixture to a boil over medium heat, then reduce the heat and let it simmer for about 10 minutes, stirring occasionally. The syrup should have a slightly thicker consistency.

10. Once the baklava is done baking, remove it from the oven, and immediately pour the hot honey syrup over the top, making sure to cover all the cuts and edges.

11. Let the baklava cool completely in the baking dish to allow the syrup to soak into the layers.

12. Once cooled, carefully remove the baklava pieces from the dish and serve them on a platter.

Variations:

- Pistachio or Almond Baklava: If you prefer other nuts, you can use pistachios or almonds instead of walnuts.

- Orange Blossom or Rose Water: To add a delightful floral touch to the honey syrup, you can substitute the fresh lemon juice with a splash of orange blossom water or rose water.

- Reduced Honey Syrup: If you want a lighter sweetness, you can reduce the amount of honey used in the syrup.

FINAL THOUGHTS AND RECOMMENDATIONS

In this Mediterranean-inspired book, we have explored the captivating world of the Mediterranean diet and its remarkable benefits for individuals living with type 2 diabetes. The journey has taken us through a culinary exploration of wholesome, flavorful, and diabetes-friendly recipes that celebrate the rich traditions and healthful practices of the Mediterranean region.

Through the lens of understanding type 2 diabetes, we have come to appreciate the significance of making mindful dietary choices. The Mediterranean Diet approach emerges as a beacon of hope, showing us that managing diabetes doesn't have to be a burdensome task.

It offers a refreshing and delicious way to nourish our bodies, uplift our spirits, and embrace a fulfilling lifestyle.

The principles and components of the Mediterranean diet reveal the essence of balanced eating, where vibrant fruits, vegetables, whole grains, legumes, and heart-healthy fats take center stage. The emphasis on fresh, locally-sourced ingredients harmonizes with the wisdom of ancient cultures, presenting us with a holistic approach to well-being.

As we delved into the scientific evidence supporting the Mediterranean diet's impact on diabetes management, we discovered compelling research validating its ability to regulate blood sugar levels, reduce the risk of complications, and even hold the potential for diabetes reversal. The long-term health benefits associated with this diet reinforce its status as a sustainable and empowering choice for individuals striving to lead healthier lives.

From Greek Yogurt Parfait with Fresh Fruits and Nuts to Turkish Baklava with Walnuts and Honey, we have explored an array of mouthwatering recipes. Each dish captures the essence of the Mediterranean diet, embracing the diverse flavors, colors, and textures that make this culinary journey so enticing. We encourage you to savor these recipes and let them inspire your creativity in the kitchen.

In the midst of this journey, we've also learned that the Mediterranean diet is not just about nourishing our bodies but fostering a sense of community and joy around the table. The act of sharing wholesome meals with loved ones nourishes not only our physical health but also our emotional well-being.

As we conclude this book, we extend our heartfelt encouragement to all readers, especially those who navigate the path of living with type 2 diabetes. Embrace the Mediterranean diet with an open heart, knowing that you hold the power to transform your relationship with food and embrace a lifestyle of vitality, balance, and joy.

Remember that small steps can lead to remarkable transformations. Embrace the Mediterranean diet one meal at a time, incorporating fresh ingredients and flavors that resonate with your taste buds and cultural preferences. Seek support from friends, family, or healthcare professionals as you embark on this journey, and remember that progress, not perfection, is the key to success.

With every meal you enjoy and every nutrient-rich ingredient you savor, you nourish not only your body but also your spirit, empowering yourself to live life to the fullest. Embrace the beauty of the Mediterranean diet, and let it become a lifelong companion on your path to better health and well-being.

May this book serve as a source of inspiration and guidance, reminding you that the power to embrace a healthier, more vibrant life resides within you. Embrace the wisdom of the Mediterranean region, and let its spirit infuse every aspect of your life. Bon appétit and savor the journey!

www.ingramcontent.com/pod-product-compliance
Lightning Source LLC
Chambersburg PA
CBHW050041260726

48658CB00005B/1705